Do

James Slavens

What You Need To Know About Doxycycline

Doxycycline is an antibiotic that can be used to treat a wide range of bacterial infections. Forms can be taken orally or injected.

Doxycycline is sometimes used by doctors to treat infections of the lungs, nose, and throat. Doxycycline can also be used to treat rosacea and acne.

Some people may not benefit from taking doxycycline. It might interface for certain different medications and can cause incidental effects. When giving doxycycline to children and pregnant women, doctors will use caution.

The numerous applications of doxycycline are examined in this article. We also talk about the warnings and side effects that doxycycline users should be aware of.

Uses

Doxycycline belongs to the tetracycline class of antibiotics. Doxycycline is prescribed by doctors for a variety of bacterial infections, including:

- lung contaminations
- physically sent contaminations (STIs)
- nose and throat contaminations
- urinary lot contaminations (UTIs)

Individuals can likewise take doxycycline in the accompanying circumstances:

Rare infections like anthrax, cholera, and typhus fever can be treated with doxycycline.

Doxycycline can be taken to prevent malaria in travelers to areas with a high risk.

Doxycycline is taken by some people to treat severe acne. The bacterium Propionibacterium acnes can cause acne, which is not an infection.

Doxycycline can be taken by people with rosacea without an antibiotic cream.

Doxycycline resistance has developed in numerous bacteria. Doctors can test the bacteria to ensure that it will respond to doxycycline before giving it to patients.

Doxycycline can be prescribed to children under the age of eight with severe or life-threatening infections if the benefits outweigh the risks.

Doryx and Doryx MPC are the brand names for doxycycline delayed-release tablets.

Doxycycline is also sold under the brand name Vibramycin, and it comes in the following forms:

Oracea is the brand name for the adult doxycycline product that doctors use to treat rosacea lesions. It comes in powder, syrup, and capsule forms.

How to take doxycycline

There are seven different forms of the antibiotic. The various forms and their strengths, expressed in milligrams (mg) or milligrams per 5 milliliters (mg/ml), are listed in the table that follows.

The delayed-release tablet Doryx MPC has a unique coating known as a modified polymer enteric coat (MPC). Doxycycline's release is slowed by 15 to 20 minutes by this coating, which is acid-resistant.

Doxycycline should be taken with a full glass of water to avoid causing irritation to the esophagus, the tube that connects the stomach to the mouth.

Doxycycline can be taken with food or milk if an esophageal irritation occurs. Doxycycline may be less absorbed by people who take it with food or milk, but this should not significantly affect the results.

Doxycycline can be used for a variety of things, and the doctor will give you a different dose for each one.

Children: Every 12 hours, a doctor will prescribe 2.2 milligrams per kilogram (mg/kg) of the child's body weight to a child weighing less than 45 kilograms (kg) with a severe or life-threatening infection. An adult dose can be given to children who weigh more than 45 kilograms.

On the first day, two doses of 4.4 mg/kg will be administered to children older than 8 years old who have less severe infections and weigh less than 45 kg. The doctor will give you two doses of 2.2 mg/kg or one dose of 2.2 mg/kg for the following days.

The adult dosage may be prescribed if the child weighs more than 45 kg and has a less serious infection.

Adults

Doctors typically prescribe 100 mg of doxycycline twice a day for adults with less serious infections on the first day, followed by 100 mg once a day. The doctor will prescribe 100 mg twice a day if the infection is severe or life-threatening.

What side effects are there?

Some people may not benefit from taking doxycycline. Doxycycline should not be taken by anyone who has had a serious reaction to it or any other tetracycline in the past.

Doxycycline may cause permanent tooth discoloration during tooth development, which occurs during the second half of pregnancy, in infancy, and childhood up to the age of eight. Teeth can take on a yellow-gray-brown hue.

When prescribing doxycycline to pregnant women or young children, doctors must weigh the potential benefits and drawbacks.

When taking doxycycline, some people may experience diarrhea caused by Clostridium difficile. This intestinal infection has the potential to be fatal or mild.

Drug interactions

Doxycycline, a member of the class of drugs known as tetracyclines, can cause bleeding.

Anticoagulants, or medications that stop blood from clotting, may need to be taken in smaller doses for some people.

Doxycycline and a penicillin antibiotic will not be prescribed by a doctor. Doxycycline prevents bacteria from growing, whereas penicillins kill bacteria. Penicillin and doxycycline may interact to prevent it from working.

The absorption of doxycycline by the body can be affected by some over-the-counter antacids, including those that contain:

- aluminum
- calcium
- magnesium
- bismuth
- subsalicylate (in Pepto Bismol)

Patients taking doxycycline may be advised to use a second method of contraception by their doctors. This is because oral contraceptives may be less effective when the antibiotic is used.

Doxycycline may interact with the following other medications:

phenytoin, barbiturates, carbamazepine, and phenytoin Doctors should get a complete medical history before giving doxycycline to patients.

Pregnancy and breastfeeding

According to the data that are currently available, researchers have concluded that therapeutic, short-term treatments with doxycycline during pregnancy are unlikely to result in abnormal birth outcomes.

Doctors will carefully prescribe doxycycline during the last half of pregnancy, particularly if the patient requires long-term use or multiple short-term courses. Doxycycline may cause yellow-gray-brown teeth discoloration in some children as they get older.

Since doxycycline can enter breast milk, breastfeeding while taking the medication could expose a child to the antibiotic. The amount of doxycycline that an infant will absorb through breast milk is unknown to researchers.

A nursing parent may receive short courses of doxycycline from their doctor. The advantages to the parent should offset the potential dangers to the newborn child. Doxycycline exposure in breast milk for an extended period of time has not been studied by researchers for its effects on infants.

Doxycycline is used to treat serious bacterial infections by doctors. Doxycycline is also used to treat acne and rosacea.

People should tell their doctors about any other medications they are taking before taking doxycycline. It's possible that taking doxycycline isn't right for everyone, especially during pregnancy. The doctor must weigh the potential risks and benefits of treatment.

Doxycycline can be taken by children as young as 8 years old, but they run the risk of having teeth that turn a permanent shade of yellow. The drug's safety or the suitability of an alternative treatment will be determined by doctors.

Cost of Doxycycline: What You Need to Know

Doxycycline is a generic drug used to treat a variety of infections, including those in children and adults. Vibramycin is one of several brand-name medications that contain doxycycline. This article provides information on the price of doxycycline as well as resources that may assist in lowering its cost.

Doxycycline can be used for:

Doxycycline is available as a tablet, capsule, or gel. It can be used to treat severe acne in adults and children, as well as to treat certain kinds of infections in adults and some children. It can also help prevent malaria in adults and some children. Additionally, it is available as an injectable solution or an oral suspension (a liquid mixture).

Check out this in-depth article for more information about doxycycline.

How much does doxycycline cost?

Doxycycline may cost you more or less. Your treatment plan, your insurance, and the pharmacy you use may all affect how much it costs. Cost may also be affected by how much you have to pay for an office visit to receive an injectable form of doxycycline.

Talk to your doctor, pharmacist, or insurance company to find out how much doxycycline will cost you.

Answers to some frequently asked questions about doxycycline's price and cost are provided below.

Does the strength or form I take affect how much doxycycline costs?

Yes, the strength or form of the medication you take can affect how much doxycycline costs. Doxycycline comes in tablet, capsule, and gel forms. Likewise accessible as an answer's given by infusion or a suspension (a fluid combination) that is taken by mouth.

The price of the drug may vary depending on its form. The price of each strength may also vary.

Keep in mind that some strengths and forms may only be available in brand-name or generic versions. Talk to your doctor or pharmacist if you want to know how much a particular brand or strength of doxycycline might cost.

What is the price of doxycycline without insurance?

Cost of doxycycline without insurance varies based on dosage and form. See "Can I get help paying for doxycycline?"

Talking to your doctor or pharmacist can also help you find out how much doxycycline might cost you without insurance. Depending on the form and strength you take, they can give you an estimate of how much you might pay for doxycycline.

Does doxycycline come in brand-name form?

Doxycycline is a brand name. It's additionally accessible in a few brand-name forms. These are some:

- Vibramycin Doryx
- Doryx MPC
- Oracea
- Acticlate
- Atridox
- Doxy 100
- Doxy 200

A generic drug is identical to a brand-name medication's active ingredient. It is believed that the generic drug is just as safe and effective as the original. Additionally, generic medications typically have lower prices than brand-name medications.

Talk to your doctor, pharmacist, or insurance provider to compare the costs of generic and brand-name doxycycline.

Talk to your doctor if you want to use brand-name doxycycline instead of the medication your doctor has prescribed. They might like one version better than the other. Additionally, you should check with your insurance company. This is due to the possibility that it will only cover one drug.

Can I get financial assistance for doxycycline?

Check out these websites if you need assistance understanding your insurance or paying for doxycycline:

NeedyMeds Medicine Assistance Tool

These websites have links to savings cards and other services, information on drug assistance programs, and information about insurance.

Talk to your doctor or pharmacist if you have any concerns regarding how to pay for doxycycline.

Which actions should I take next?

Talk to your doctor or pharmacist if you still have questions about the cost of doxycycline. They might be able to give you a better idea of how much this drug will cost. However, if you have health insurance, you will need to talk to your insurance company to find out how much doxycycline will actually cost you.

You might want to ask your doctor or insurance company the following questions:

Will the amount of doxycycline I take affect how much it costs?

Might my measurement at any point be changed in light of which type of doxycycline I can manage?

Are there alternative treatments for my condition that might be less expensive?

If I can't afford my medication, what should I do?

Subscribe to any of Healthline's newsletters to learn about various conditions and health improvement tips. You may likewise need to look at the internet based networks at Bezzy. It is a location where individuals with particular conditions can connect with others and receive assistance.

Highlights of Doxycycline

Doxycycline oral tablet can be purchased as a generic as well as a brand-name medication. Brands like: Doryx, Acticlate, and Doryx MPC

Doxycycline can be taken orally in three forms: a suspension, a capsule, and a tablet. Additionally, it comes as an injection solution that can only be administered by a healthcare professional.

The oral tablet doxycycline is used to treat severe acne and infections. Additionally, it prevents malaria.

Side effects of doxycycline

The oral tablet of doxycycline can cause side effects. Some are more prevalent, while others are serious.

Doxycycline's most common side effects can include the following:

Appetite loss, nausea, and vomiting, diarrhea, hives, sun sensitivity, and temporary discoloration of adult teeth (which goes away when the drug is stopped by the dentist). If these effects are mild, they may pass in a few days or a few weeks. Talk to your pharmacist or doctor if they become more severe or persist.

This medication does not make you sleepy.

Serious side effects

If you experience serious side effects, talk to your doctor right away. If you think you are experiencing a medical emergency or if your symptoms appear to be life-threatening, dial 911. The following are examples of serious side effects and how they can be felt:

Diarrhea brought on by antibiotics

Some of the signs include:

Bloody diarrhea, severe diarrhea, stomach cramps, pain, fever, dehydration, loss of appetite, and weight loss are all symptoms of severe diarrhea. Some of the signs include:

Headache, double vision, vision loss, irritation of the esophagus, or esophageal ulcers (may be more likely if you take your medication at night). Some of the signs include:

- chest pain or burning
- Anemia
- Pancreatitis

Some of the signs include:

severe skin reactions, such as pain in your upper abdomen or pain in your abdomen that moves to your back or gets worse after eating fever Some of the signs include:

blisters, peeling skin, and a rash of tiny purple spots

Our objective is to offer you the most current and pertinent information. We cannot, however, guarantee that this information covers all possible side effects due to the fact that different people react differently to drugs. Do not rely solely on this information for medical advice. Always talk to a healthcare professional who knows your medical history about potential side effects.

Important warnings about permanent tooth color changes: If given to children while they are still developing their teeth, this medication may cause permanent changes in the color of their teeth. This spans from the last half of a pregnancy to the age of eight. Teeth in children can turn yellow, gray, or brown.

Warning about diarrhea brought on by antibiotics: Diarrhea linked to antibiotics may occur with this medication. This can be anything from mild diarrhea to a serious colon infection. This effect can, in rare instances, result in death. Inform your doctor if you experience severe or persistent diarrhea. They might stop giving you this drug.

Alert for intracranial hypertension: High blood pressure within your skull, or intracranial hypertension, may result from this medication. Headaches, double vision, blurry vision, and vision loss are all possible signs. If you experience any of these symptoms, see a doctor right away. Additionally, you may have swelling in your eyes. This condition is more common in overweight women who are pregnant. Your risk is also higher if you have had intracranial hypertension in the past.

Warning for severe skin reactions: Skin reactions can be severe with this medication. Stevens-Johnson syndrome, toxic epidermal necrolysis, and the drug reaction with eosinophilia and systemic symptoms (DRESS) are examples of these. Side effects can incorporate rankles, stripping skin, and a rash of little purple spots. Stop taking this medication and contact your doctor right away if you experience any of these symptoms.

Delay in bone growth that is reversible: If the mother takes this medication during the second and third trimesters of pregnancy, it may prevent children's bone growth. If taken by children under the age of eight, it may also stop them from growing bones. When the medication is stopped, this delayed bone growth can be reversed.

Warning about photosensitivity: Your skin may become more sensitive to sunlight than usual as a result of this medication. A skin rash, itching, redness, or severe sunburn may result from brief exposure to sunlight. If you are taking this medication, try to avoid the sun. Wear protective clothing and apply sunscreen if you can't.

Doxycycline: what is it?

Acticlate, Doryx, and Doryx MPC are all brands of the prescription medication doxycycline oral tablet. Generic versions of it are also available. Usually, generic drugs cost less. They might not always be available in the same strength or form as the brand-name version in all cases.

There are immediate-release and delayed-release doxycycline tablets available. Doxycycline can also be taken orally in two other forms: solution and a capsule. Doxycycline also comes in an injection solution that can only be given by a medical professional.

Doxycycline is prescribed to treat bacterial infections. Skin infections, eye infections, respiratory infections, and other infections can all fall under this category. It is also used to treat severe acne as an additional treatment and to prevent malaria in travelers to malaria-prone areas.

In combination therapy, this medication may be used. Because of this, you might have to take it with other medications.

How it Works

Doxycycline is a member of the tetracycline class of drugs. A group of drugs with similar effects is called a class of drugs. Similar conditions are frequently treated with these medications.

By preventing the production of a bacterial protein, this medication works. By binding to specific parts of the protein, it accomplishes this. This treats your infection and stops the protein from growing.

Other medications, vitamins, and herbs may interact with Doxycycline. Doxycycline oral tablet can interact with other medications, vitamins, and herbs. When a substance alters the way a drug works, this is called an interaction. This may be harmful or hinder the drug's effectiveness.

Your doctor should carefully manage all of your medications to help prevent interactions. Make certain to enlighten your primary care physician concerning all meds, nutrients, or spices you're taking. Talk to your doctor or pharmacist about how this medication might interact with other medications you are taking.

The following is a list of drugs that might interact with doxycycline.

Drugs that shouldn't be taken with doxycycline

You shouldn't take these drugs with doxycycline. This could have harmful effects on your body. Drugs like these are examples:

Penicillin.

Doxycycline may hinder penicillin's ability to kill bacteria.

Isotretinoin.

Doxycycline and isotretinoin can increase your risk of intracranial hypertension when taken together.

Drug-drug interactions that may reduce their effectiveness

When taken with other medications, doxycycline may not be as effective in treating your condition. This is because there may be less doxycycline in your body. This kind of interaction can be caused by drugs like:

Preparations containing bismuth subsalicylate, aluminum, calcium, magnesium, and iron Antacids Seizure medications like barbiturates, carbamazepine, and phenytoin Interactions that can increase side effects Taking doxycycline with certain medications increases your risk of experiencing side effects from these medications. Examples of drugs that might interact this way include:

<u>Warfarin.</u>

If you need to take warfarin with doxycycline, your doctor may reduce the dose.

Warnings Regarding Doxycycline

The Doxycycline oral tablet comes with a number of warnings.

Warning about Doxycycline's potential to trigger severe allergic reactions

Some of the signs include:

breathing difficulties swelling of the tongue or throat If you experience an allergic reaction, you should immediately contact your doctor or the poison control center in your area. Call 911 or go to the nearest ER if your symptoms are severe.

If you have ever experienced an allergic reaction to this medication or any other tetracyclines, do not take it again. The second dose could result in death.

Warning about interactions with other foods

Calcium-rich foods may prevent your body from absorbing this medication. As a result, it might not be as effective at treating your condition. Milk and cheese are two examples of foods high in calcium. At least one hour before or one hour after taking this medication, avoid these foods and beverages.

Precautions for individuals with particular health conditions In the case of overweight women who are pregnant: This medication increases your risk of developing high blood pressure within your skull. If this medication is right for you, ask your doctor.

For people who have had intracranial hypertension in the past: This medication increases your risk of developing high blood pressure within your skull. If this medication is right for you, ask your doctor.

Other groups that should be aware of: Pregnant women Doxycycline's use during pregnancy has not been adequately studied.

Converse with your primary care physician on the off chance that you're pregnant or intending to become pregnant. You should inquire of your physician regarding the specific risk to the pregnancy. If the drug's potential benefits outweigh the potential risk to the pregnancy, only then should it be used. If you become pregnant while taking this medication, immediately contact your doctor.

For ladies who are breastfeeding: Doxycycline can pass into a baby's breast milk and can have side effects on a baby who is breastfed. If you breastfeed your child, talk to your doctor about it. You might have to decide whether to stop taking this medication or stop breastfeeding.

Senior adults: It's possible that older people's kidneys aren't working as well as they used to. Your body may process drugs more slowly as a result of this. As a result, your body absorbs more of the drug over time. This makes you more likely to get side effects.

For youngsters: During the period of tooth development, this drug may cause tooth discoloration.

Children under the age of eight should not be given this medication unless the potential benefits outweigh the risks. When no other treatments are available or have been demonstrated to be effective, its use in these children is recommended for the treatment of severe or life-threatening conditions like anthrax or Rocky Mountain spotted fever.

How to Take Doxycycline

This dosage information applies to oral tablets of Doxycycline. This may not cover all possible drug forms and dosages. Your measurements, drug structure, and how frequently you take the medication will rely upon:

your age, the condition that is being treated, how severe it is, any other medical conditions you have, and how you react to the first dose. The dosage information below is for the conditions that are most frequently prescribed for this drug. It's possible that not all conditions for which this medication can be prescribed by your doctor are on this list. Talk to your doctor if you have any questions about your prescription.

Generic forms and strengths:

Form of Doxycycline:

Form: 20 mg, 50 mg, 75 mg, 100 mg, and 150 mg strengths of an oral tablet: oral delayed-release tablet

Benefits: 50, 75, 100, 150, and 200 milligrams Brand:

Form of Action: strengths of an oral tablet: 150 mg, 75 mg, and 150 mg

Form of Doryx: oral delayed-release tablet

Benefits: 50, 75, 80, 100, 150, and 200 milligrams

Brand: Form for Doryx MPC: postponed discharge oral tablet

Strength: Adult dose of 120 milligrams for infection: Generic immediate-release:

Common dosages: 200 mg taken once daily for the first 12 hours of treatment. The next dose is 100 mg per day. 100 mg every 12 hours is suggested for more severe infections.

Acticlate and Doryx:

Common dosages: 200 mg taken once daily for the first 12 hours of treatment. The next dose is 100 mg, which can be taken once daily or 50 mg every 12 hours. For additional serious diseases, 100 mg like clockwork is suggested.

MPC of Doryx:

Common dosages: 120 mg every 12 hours for a total of 240 mg on the first day of treatment. The next dose is 120 mg, which can be taken once daily or 60 mg every 12 hours. 120 mg every 12 hours is suggested for more severe infections.

Dosage for children ages 8 to 17: Acticlate and generic immediate-release:

For children who have a severe or life-threatening infection like Rocky Mountain spotted fever and weigh less than 45 kilograms: Every 12 hours, take 2.2 mg/kg as directed.

For children who are older than 8 years, weigh less than 99 pounds (45 kilograms), and have a less severe infection: On the first day of treatment, the dosage of 4.4 mg/kg, divided into two doses, is recommended. From that point forward, the day to day support measurements ought to be 2.2 mg/kg, given as a solitary portion or isolated into two everyday dosages.

For children weighing at least 45 kilograms (99 pounds): Concentrate on adults.

Doryx:

Children under the age of 9 who weigh less than or equal to 45 kg: On the first day of treatment, the recommended dosage is 4.4 mg/kg divided into two doses. The next dose is 2.2 mg/kg, which can be taken as a single daily dose or divided into two.

For an infection that is worse: It is possible to use doses up to 4.4 mg/kg.

For children who weigh more than 45 kilograms (99 pounds): Concentrate on adults.

MPC of Doryx:

For children who have a severe or life-threatening infection like Rocky Mountain spotted fever and weigh less than 45 kilograms: Every 12 hours, a dose of 2.6 mg/kg is recommended.

For children who are older than 8 years, weigh less than 99 pounds (45 kilograms), and have a less severe infection: On the first day of treatment, the dosage of 5.3 mg/kg, divided into two doses, is recommended. After that, a single dose of 2.6 mg/kg or two daily doses should be taken as the daily maintenance dose.

For children weighing at least 45 kilograms (99 pounds): Concentrate on adults.

Youngster dose (ages 0-7 years)

It has not been affirmed that this medication is protected and compelling for use in individuals who are more youthful than 8 years.

Dosage for seniors (over 65)

Your doctor may start you on a different schedule or a lower dose. This can help prevent your body's levels of this drug from getting too high.

Adult doses for malaria prevention consist of generic immediate-release, Doryx, and Acticlate:

Common dosages: 100 mg per day. Start treatment one to two days before going to a malaria-endemic area. After leaving the area, continue the daily treatment for four weeks.

MPC of Doryx:

Common dosages: 120 mg per day Start treatment one to two days before going to a malaria-endemic area. Proceed with day to day treatment for quite some time in the wake of leaving the region.

Dosage for children (ages 8 to 17): Doryx, Acticlate, and generic immediate-release medications

Common dosages: 2 mg/kg once daily up to the dose for adults. Start treatment one to two days before going to a malaria-endemic area. After leaving the area, continue the daily treatment for four weeks.

MPC of Doryx:

Common dosages: up to the adult dose of 2.4 mg/kg once daily. Start treatment one to two days before going to a malaria-endemic area. After leaving the area, continue the daily treatment for four weeks.

Dosage for children (ages 0–7)

It has not been proven that this medication is safe or effective for children younger than 8 years old.

Dosage for seniors (over 65)

Your doctor may start you on a different schedule or a lower dose. This can help prevent your body's levels of this drug from getting too high.

Doxycycline oral tablets are taken as directed for short-term treatment. If you don't take it as directed, you run the risk of serious side effects.

If you suddenly stop taking the medication or don't take any at all: It's likely that your infection won't go away. You won't be protected from certain infections if you take it to prevent malaria. It could be fatal.

If you don't take the medication as directed or miss doses: It's possible that your medication won't work as well or won't work at all. You might feel quite a bit improved before you follow through with your course of treatment, however you ought to continue to accept your drug as coordinated. Your treatment may not work as well if you miss doses or don't finish the entire course. Antibiotic resistance may also result. This indicates that doxycycline and other antibiotics will not treat your infection in the future.

If you consume in excess: You run the risk of having dangerous levels of the drug in your body and developing additional adverse effects. Call your doctor or the poison control center in your area if you think you have taken too much of this medication. Call 911 right away or go to the nearest emergency room if your symptoms are severe.

If you miss a dose, what should you do? As soon as you remember, take your medication. Take only one dose if you remember less than an hour before your next scheduled dose. Do not attempt to catch up by taking two doses simultaneously. This could lead to harmful side effects.

How to determine whether the drug is working: You might feel better and your symptoms might start to get better.

Important things to keep in mind before taking doxycycline

Keep these things in mind if your doctor gives you an oral tablet of doxycycline.

The oral tablet can be cut, but it should not be crushed. You can take this medication with or without food. You can break up the delayed-release tablet and sprinkle it on applesauce if you are unable to swallow it whole. Consume the mixture immediately without chewing.

Storage Store this medication between 69°F and 77°F (20°C and 25°C) at room temperature.

Keep this drug out of direct sunlight.

This medication should not be stored in bathrooms or other moist or damp areas.

Take your medication with you when you travel:

Always keep your medications close by. Never put it in a checked bag while flying. It should be kept in your carry-on bag.

Don't worry about the x-ray machines at the airport. Your medication will not be harmed by them.

It's possible that you'll need to show the airport staff your medication's label. Keep the original prescription-labeled box with you at all times.

Do not leave this medication in your car or in the glove compartment. Avoid doing this when it is extremely hot or extremely cold.

Sensitivity to the sun This medication may make your skin more sensitive to the sun and raise your risk of getting burned by it. If possible, avoid the sun. Wear protective clothing and apply sunscreen if you can't.

Insurance: This drug requires prior authorization from many insurance companies. This indicates that before your insurance company will pay for the prescription, your doctor may need to obtain approval from them.

Do you have any other options?

You can treat your condition with other medications. Some might suit you better than others. Discuss with your doctor other medication options that might be effective for you.

Can dairy products be consumed while taking doxycycline?

Doxycycline is an anti-microbial. It can also be used to prevent malaria and treat a wide range of bacterial infections. Dairy products can affect the effectiveness of doxycycline when consumed with it.

In this article, we'll take a closer look at how dairy products and other substances can make doxycycline less effective.

What is doxycycline and how does it work?

Tetracyclines are a group of antibiotics that include doxycycline. By stopping bacteria from making proteins, these antibiotics work. Bacteria are unable to develop or flourish as a result.

Doxycycline can be purchased as a tablet, capsule, or liquid. Tablets and capsules with a delayed release are also available.

The following conditions may be treated with this medication:

Dental infections, flea and tick bites, intestinal infections, lung infections, sexually transmitted infections, adult acne caused by rosacea, arthritis caused by Lyme disease, skin infections, throat infections, and urinary tract infections can all be treated with this medication.

Additionally, doxycycline may be prescribed to prevent additional complications following exposure to the anthrax bacteria.

Can dairy products diminish its efficiency?

Dairy products like milk, cheese, and yogurt can make it harder for your body to absorb doxycycline. This is especially true if you take this medication at the same time as dairy products.

This is because dairy products contain calcium. Calcium ions react with doxycycline in a process called chelation to create a new chemical compound called a chelate. Your gastrointestinal tract absorbs less doxycycline as a result.

Calcium-containing antacids and supplements may have a similar effect. Doxycycline also chelates when it comes into contact with other nutrients from food, like iron and magnesium.

The extent to which calcium chelation affects doxycycline's overall efficacy is unknown. Even though there is only a slight effect, it is still a good idea to avoid dairy products while you are taking doxycycline.

When are dairy products safe to eat?

Dairy products can usually be consumed safely two hours before or after taking doxycycline.

Within two hours of taking doxycycline, you should avoid certain common dairy products, including:

Desserts made with dairy products, as well as milk, buttermilk, cheese, butter cream, ice cream, cottage cheese, cream cheese, sour cream, ghee, kefir, condensed milk yogurt, and frozen yogurt, as well as whey and whey protein

Doxycycline can interact with a number of other substances, including dairy products. Some examples include:

Antibiotics, antacids, anticoagulants (blood thinners), anticonvulsants, antimetabolites, barbiturates, diuretics, iron supplements, laxatives, lithium, proton pump inhibitors, retinoids, vitamin A supplements, and others Your doctor will be able to use this information to figure out the safest way for you to take doxycycline.

Doxycycline can also interact with alcohol. Although it is generally safe to drink in moderation, you should discuss your usual alcohol consumption with your doctor.

Lastly, birth control pills, patches, vaginal rings, injections, and implants can be rendered less effective by doxycycline. If you must take doxycycline, talk to your doctor about other methods of contraception.

Are most people safe from it?

The majority of adults and children over the age of 12 can take doxycycline safely. It's not suggested during pregnancy or while nursing.

If you've ever experienced any of the following, tell your doctor.

Asthma, drug allergies, esophagitis, intracranial hypertension, kidney disease, liver disease, lupus myasthenia gravis, and an oral or vaginal yeast infection can all affect the stomach.

How to take doxycycline safely and effectively

Follow the prescription label carefully. When taking delayed-release tablets or capsules, do not crush, chew, split, or open them.

Doxycycline pills should be taken with a glass of water. Consult your doctor or pharmacist for alternatives if you are unable to swallow the pill.

Make sure to drink a lot of water after taking doxycycline. Avoid lying down because the pill may become entangled in your esophagus, causing irritation.

If you miss a dose, take it as soon as you remember, unless your next dose is almost due. To make up for a missed dose, do not take two doses at once.

Complete the medication regimen. Even if your symptoms subside after a few days, it is essential to take all of the medication that was prescribed to you. Symptoms may return if you stop taking doxycycline too soon. Resistance to antibiotics can also develop. Additionally, you ought to try not to take doxycycline for longer than demonstrated.

Cover your skin whenever you can, wear a hat, and apply sunscreen. Your skin may become more sensitive to sunlight after taking doxycycline.

How to take doxycycline to prevent malaria When you take doxycycline to prevent malaria, you must begin taking it one to two days before traveling to a malaria-endemic region. You are required to continue taking it while you are there and for the subsequent four weeks. Doxycycline for malaria should not be taken for more than four months in total.

Additionally, keep in mind that doxycycline is not 100% effective for malaria prevention. To avoid mosquitoes, it's important to take other precautions. This means using an insect repellent, covering up, staying inside, especially at night and dawn.

Doxycycline is an antibiotic that belongs to the tetracycline class and is used to treat infections in the skin, eyes, mouth, lungs, and many other parts of the body. Additionally, it prevents malaria.

Calcium, which can interact with doxycycline, can be found in dairy products. A chemical reaction occurs when these two substances come into contact, which can reduce the amount of doxycycline absorbed by the body. Doxycycline may become less effective as a result.

Avoid eating dairy products within two hours of taking a dose of doxycycline to ensure its effectiveness. For additional guidance on how to safely take doxycycline, consult your physician or pharmacist.

Can Doxycycline be taken with alcohol?

While taking doxycycline, most people can have one or two drinks on occasion, but people who drink a lot might want to try another antibiotic. Doxycycline could be less effective if you drink a lot.

Doxycycline is an antibiotic used to treat respiratory and skin infections among other bacterial infections. Additionally, it is used to prevent malaria, a parasitic disease spread by mosquitoes.

Antibiotics come in a variety of varieties, or classes. Doxycycline is in the antibiotic medication class, which impedes microbes' capacity to make proteins. Bacteria can't expand and thrive in this way.

Several antibiotics, including doxycycline, can interact with alcohol in some cases.

Can I have a drink?

If a person has a long or heavy alcohol use history, doxycycline may interact with alcohol.

This condition is defined by the National Institute on Alcohol Abuse and Alcoholism as drinking more than four drinks per day for men and three drinks per day for women.

Doxycycline and alcohol can also interact with liver problems.

Drinking alcohol while taking doxycycline can make the antibiotic less effective in these two groups.

However, if you are taking doxycycline and are not exposed to these dangers, you should be able to consume one or two drinks without compromising the antibiotic's effectiveness.

What will occur if I consume alcohol?

Metronidazole and tinidazole, two antibiotics, have serious interactions with alcohol that can cause a variety of side effects, such as:

Drowsiness

Drowsiness in the stomach, nausea, vomiting, headache, and rapid heart rate. Drinking one or two alcoholic beverages while taking doxycycline shouldn't cause any of these side effects.

However, if you are still recovering from an infection, avoid alcohol. According to Trusted Source, drinking alcohol, particularly a lot of it, can affect how well your immune system works.

According to research, taking doxycycline with alcohol lowers doxycycline levels in the blood and may have an impact on its effectiveness. After quitting drinking, the effects can last for days.

The manufacturer suggests substituting drugs for alcohol for those who are likely to drink.

What if I've had a few drinks already?

If you have been drinking and are taking doxycycline, don't drink any more, especially if you notice any of the following:

Dizziness, Drowsiness, and Stomach upset are not serious side effects of taking doxycycline with alcohol. However, overindulging in alcohol can have a negative impact on your recovery.

Drinking alcohol can slow your body's immune response for up to 24 hours, according to the National Institute on Alcohol Abuse and Alcoholism.

It's also important to remember that drinking alcohol may make it more likely for people to fall, which could cause bleeding, especially if they're older or on blood thinners.

Is there anything else I should avoid while taking doxycycline?

Any medications or supplements you take, including herbal or over-the-counter ones, should always be reported to your doctor.

Be sure to check with your doctor before taking doxycycline:

Barbiturates, anticoagulants, anticonvulsants like carbamazepine and phenytoin, diuretics like lithium methotrexate, proton pump inhibitors, retinoid, vitamin A supplements, and Tetracycline antibiotics like doxycycline can also make you more sensitive to sunlight. Bismuth subsalicylate is an active ingredient in medications like Pepto-Bismol. When you go outside, protect yourself from the sun by covering up with protective clothing and applying a lot of sunscreen.

Doxycycline should not be taken by pregnant women, women who are nursing, or children under the age of 8.

In conclusion, a number of bacterial infections can be treated with Doxycycline, an antibiotic.

While it can be risky to drink alcohol while taking some antibiotics, it is generally safe to drink alcohol occasionally while taking doxycycline.

Doxycycline should not be taken while a person is taking multiple medications, has a liver condition, or is a chronic drinker.

Remember that liquor can dial back your body's resistant reaction. If you decide to drink while taking doxycycline, your recovery from the underlying infection may take an additional day.

Combining Alcohol and Antibiotics: Is It Risky?

Your risk of experiencing side effects can rise if you take antibiotics with alcohol. It is best to avoid drinking alcohol until you have completed your course of antibiotics.

Drugs and alcohol can be dangerous together. While taking a variety of drugs, doctors advise avoiding alcohol.

The most pressing concern is that taking medications with alcohol may raise the likelihood of dangerous side effects.

In this section, we'll talk about how safe it is to mix antibiotics and alcohol. Additionally, we'll talk about how alcohol can affect your body's ability to fight infections.

Can I consume alcohol with antibiotics?

Interactions

While drinking alcohol does not reduce the effectiveness of the majority of antibiotics, it may increase your risk of experiencing certain side effects, particularly if you consume an excessive amount.

When you are taking any of the following antibiotics, you should never drink alcohol:

Taking cefoperazone, cefotetan, metronidazole, ketoconazole, isoniazid, linezolid, and griseofulvin with alcohol can result in a potentially harmful reaction.

Tinidazole, cefotetan, ketoconazole, metronidazole, and cefoperazone can all be caused by drinking alcohol while taking these medications:

Drinking alcohol before, during, or up to three days after taking these drugs may cause nausea, vomiting, flushing, headache, rapid heartbeat, and stomach cramps.

Griseofulvin When taking this medication, consuming alcohol can result in:

flushing, excessive sweating, and a rapid heartbeat are side effects of isoniazid and linezolid. Taking these medications with alcohol can cause side effects such as:

Doxycycline and erythromycin can cause liver damage and high blood pressure. If you drink alcohol while taking these antibiotics, they may be less effective.

Side effects of the drug in general

The specific side effects that an antibiotic can cause vary from drug to drug. Antibiotics, on the other hand, frequently cause the following side effects:

Constipation, drowsiness, dizziness, lightheadedness, and diarrhea can all be brought on by alcohol. These are some:

a bloated stomach, digestive issues like stomach pain, diarrhea, and ulcers, and fatigue are all indicators of a negative alcohol-antibiotic reaction.

severe headache, rapid heart rate, and flushing (skin reddening and warming) are the most common side effects. Immediately dial 911 or your local emergency services number if you think you are experiencing a medical emergency.

What to Do

Your antibiotic's warning label ought to include information about drinking.

If you have any questions about the specifics of your medications, speak with your doctor or pharmacist. They might tell you that having a drink now and then is fine. However, this is probably contingent on your age, general health, and the kind of medication you are taking.

Ask your doctor how long you should wait before drinking again if your doctor says you shouldn't.

Before drinking alcohol, you may need to wait at least 72 hours after finishing your antibiotic treatment.

You can avoid alcohol-drug interactions by following your doctor's or pharmacist's instructions.

Effects of alcohol on infection healing

In most cases, drinking alcohol will not prevent your antibiotic from working to treat your infection. However, there are other ways in which it can hinder the healing of your infection.

You can recover from illness or infection by getting enough rest and eating well. Alcohol can affect these factors in a negative way.

Drinking alcohol, for instance, can disrupt your sleeping patterns. It might prevent you from sleeping well at night.

Your body may also be prevented from absorbing essential nutrients by alcohol. It has the potential to drain your energy and raise your blood sugar levels.

Your body's ability to recover from an infection can be hindered by any one of these factors. It doesn't matter if you take medication or not—acute, binge, and chronic alcohol use can all be harmful.

Keep in mind that alcoholic beverages include more than just liquor, beer, wine, and mixed drinks. It is also present in some mouthwashes and cold medicines.

If you have ever experienced an adverse reaction to alcohol or antibiotics, check the ingredient labels of these and other products. Ask your doctor if using these items while taking an antibiotic is safe.

Antibiotics are frequently prescribed by doctors for a short time. To fully recover from an infection, you typically only need to take antibiotics for a week or two.

Consult your doctor before taking antibiotics and alcohol together. Both alcohol and antibiotics can have negative effects on the body, and taking antibiotics while drinking alcohol can make it more likely that you will experience these negative effects.

Follow the instructions on your medication's label to avoid alcohol consumption during treatment.

Remember that anti-toxins are much of the time endorsed on a momentary premise. Consider delaying your next drink until you stop taking your medications. It might lessen the likelihood of antibiotic-related problems or side effects.

You will probably be able to get over your infection more quickly if you don't drink alcohol.

If you are taking an antibiotic, tell your doctor and pharmacist. They can talk to you about your medications and alcohol use.

What negative effects do antibiotics have?

Antibiotics are prescribed by medical professionals to treat and prevent bacterial infections. The majority of antibiotic-related side effects are not life-threatening. However, some people may experience severe side effects from antibiotics that necessitate medical attention.

Most of the time, antibiotics are safe, and doctors give them to stop bacteria from growing; for instance, to treat urinary tract infections (UTIs), skin infections, and bacterial infections like strep throat.

The majority of upper respiratory infections, the common cold, and COVID-19 are not treatable with antibiotics.

However, antibiotic-related side effects can range from mild to severe to potentially fatal. Antibiotic side effects account for one in five emergency room visits, according to the Centers for Disease Control and Prevention (CDC).

A medical professional should be consulted by anyone experiencing severe antibiotic side effects. Call 911 if you notice any of the symptoms of anaphylaxis, such as difficulty breathing, chest pain, or tightness in the throat.

Antibiotics' common and uncommon side effects, as well as long-term side effects and when to see a doctor, are discussed in this article.

Here are more facts about bacteria.

Antibiotic-related side effects Common side effects include:

Issues with the digestive system Common digestive symptoms include:

stomach pain or cramping, nausea, indigestion, vomiting, diarrhea, fullness, and loss of appetite are all symptoms of indigestion. Sometimes they have to take them with nothing to eat. The best way to take an antibiotic can be discussed with a doctor or pharmacist.

When an individual stops taking the antibiotic, the majority of their digestive issues go away.

Stop taking antibiotics right away if you experience digestive side effects like bloody diarrhea, severe abdominal pain, or uncontrollable vomiting.

Here, you can learn more about other common digestive issues.

Infection caused by fungi

Antibiotics kill harmful bacteria. However, they occasionally disrupt the natural balance of the body's natural flora and kill the beneficial bacteria that guard against fungal infections.

Antibiotic use can result in a fungal (candida) infection of the mouth, digestive tract, or vagina as a result of this imbalance.

Thrush is another name for candidiasis in the mouth and throat.

Thrush can cause the following symptoms:

white patches on the throat, cheeks, roof of the mouth, or tongue; pain while eating or swallowing; bleeding when brushing teeth; and fungal infections are typically treated with antifungal medications like nystatin.

Here, you can learn more about the gut microbiota.

Antibiotics for UTIs and yeast infections Treating a UTI with antibiotics can occasionally result in a yeast infection in the vaginal area.

A vaginal yeast infection may exhibit the following symptoms:

pain and a burning sensation in the vaginal area during sexual activity and when urinating abdominal or pelvic pain blood in the urine white to gray lumpy discharge from the vaginal area fever and chills Doctors frequently prescribe fluconazole to treat yeast infections brought on by UTI antibiotics.

13472598R00037